FOR PARENTS OF A CHILD NEWLY-DIAGNOSED WITH TYPE 1 DIABETES

Dennis Gooler, PhD

Susan Guzman, PhD

Dynamic Diabetes Solutions

San Diego, California

2014

Copyright, authors and disclaimer

E-Booklet Title	For Parents of a Child Newly-Diagnosed with Type 1 Diabetes
Authors	Dennis D. Gooler, PhD
	Susan Guzman, PhD
Copyright	Copyright @ 2014. All rights reserved.
Publisher	Dynamic Diabetes Solutions
Contact	Dr. Dennis Gooler
	Dynamic Diabetes Solutions
	12091 Tretagnier Circle
	San Diego, CA 92128
	858-776-8452
	dgooler@gmail.com

Disclaimer

Dynamic Diabetes Solutions does not provide medical advice, diagnoses, or treatment for any form of diabetes or complications that may result from diabetes.

- This e-booklet contains general information about medical conditions and treatments pertaining to diabetes. The information is not medical advice, and should not be treated as such.
- You must not rely on the information in this e-booklet as an alternative to medical advice from your doctor or other professional healthcare provider.
- If you have any specific questions about any medical matter you should consult your doctor or other professional healthcare provider.
- The information in this e-booklet is for educational purposes only.

Content in E-Booklets from Dynamic Diabetes Solutions

E-booklets prepared by Dynamic Diabetes Solutions feature original writing and *aggregated information.* By aggregated information, we mean information that has been gleaned from a variety of credible web sites, and summarized as appropriate to enhance the points being made in each e-booklet.

Information referenced in this document is taken from sources that are generally readily available to the reader. Only rarely will information from a journal or other print source, not easily available to the reader, be cited. Reference to the source of previously published material is clearly identified and, insofar as possible, the URL address is provided in the reference list at the end of this booklet.

Because this e-booklet contains references to specific web sites, the authors recognize that web sites change, come, and go. All URLs identified in this e-booklet were active at the time of writing. However, it is possible that a particular web site may disappear, or be significantly altered. Therefore, advance warning is given that some web sites links may no longer be operating. Such is the nature of our very fluid Internet world.

Many people with diabetes, or those who care from them could, with enough time and effort, find many of the internet resources we cite on their own. But we find most people with diabetes have neither the time nor the inclination to conduct exhaustive searches on the web when what they need is targeted information, and they need it now!

The primary service Dynamic Diabetes Solutions provides through these e-booklets is to help readers gain access quickly and easily to information from a variety of credible sources, on a given topic.

We trust these e-booklets will be of assistance in that regard.

The Shock of Diagnosis

The experts agree: finding out that your child has type 1 diabetes comes as a shock to most parents:

> If you're like most parents who have just been told your child or teen has type 1 diabetes, it is a complete shock. Only about 10 percent of the time do we find a family history of type 1 diabetes. [1]

> A diagnosis of diabetes can send shock waves through your entire family. It will take some time for your family to work through all the emotions that started with the diagnosis-- but it will happen. Caring for diabetes will simply become a part of family life. But in the first weeks and months after diagnosis, expect that you, your child, and your family will experience an array of emotions. [2]

> As a parent of a child with diabetes, the diagnosis can often be a much harder blow for the parent than for the child. Your child's diagnosis will likely come as a great shock and it can be difficult to recognize just how much of an effect it can have on you. [3]

Parents whose children have been diagnosed with type 1 diabetes speak eloquently about the shock:

> *"All of a sudden, my face felt flushed and the doctor's words sounded foreign, like she must have been talking to somebody else. Tony and I kept looking at each other, then at John and then shifting our eyes to the doctor and nurses again. Our questions started flowing and the whole world changed for our perfect little boy. I started thinking about how many changes we would expect him to make. How many challenges he would face ... how different he seemed just one week ago. What we were hearing swirled above us like cartoon birdies once you've been hit on the head."* [4]

> *"D-DAY, TUESDAY, DECEMBER 14, 1999, approximately 4:00 p.m. I came out of the department store and checked the voice mail on my cell phone immediately to see if my wife, Toni, had called concerning the result of our daughter Megan's doctor's appointment. There were five messages. I didn't need to listen to them. Five messages could only mean one thing ... my daughter had diabetes. I couldn't listen to the messages at first. I had to try to compose myself for what I knew was coming. I started to cry. All the usual thoughts started to go through my mind ... what terrible sin had I committed to deserve this, why my daughter, why my family, how could a good father allow this to happen to his daughter, wasn't it my duty as a father to protect my daughter?"* [5]

"When the doctors told me and my wife that our daughter Arden had type I diabetes, I broke down and sobbed uncontrollably. I found it impossible to look my wife Kelly in the face, I didn't want her to see me so destroyed and I definitely couldn't find it within myself to witness her heart breaking. The days, weeks and months that followed felt otherworldly, my head was ringing and I constantly felt like someone had reached down my throat and was strangling my heart. I struggled at times to look Arden in the eyes for fear that I would cry." [6]

What is type 1 diabetes?

When your child was diagnosed with type 1 diabetes, you were no doubt given information about the disease. However, since most parents are in a state of shock when they receive the diagnosis, it is possible you may not remember all the information your health care team gave you about type 1 diabetes. To refresh your memory, here are some descriptions of type 1:

The American Diabetes Association offers this description of type 1 diabetes:

> Type 1 diabetes is usually diagnosed in children and young adults, and was previously known as juvenile diabetes. Only 5% of people with diabetes have this form of the disease. In type 1 diabetes, the body

does not produce insulin. Insulin is a hormone that is needed to convert sugar, starches and other food into energy needed for daily life. With the help of insulin therapy and other treatments, even young children can learn to manage their condition and live long, healthy lives. [7]

The Diabetes Research Institute Foundation offers this explanation of type 1 diabetes:

The more severe form of diabetes is type 1, or insulin-dependent diabetes. It's sometimes called "juvenile" diabetes, because type 1 diabetes usually develops in children and teenagers, though it can develop at any age.

With type 1 diabetes, the body's immune system attacks part of its own pancreas. Scientists are not sure why. But the immune system mistakenly sees the insulin-producing cells in the pancreas as foreign, and destroys them. This attack is known as "autoimmune" disease.

These cells – called "islets" (pronounced EYE-lets) – are the ones that sense glucose in the blood and, in response, produce the necessary amount of insulin to normalize blood sugars. Insulin serves as a "key" to open your cells, to allow the glucose to enter

-- and allow you to use the glucose for energy.

Without insulin, there is no "key." So, the sugar stays -- and builds up-- in the blood. The result: the body's cells starve from the lack of glucose.

And, if left untreated, the high level of "blood sugar" can damage eyes, kidneys, nerves, and the heart, and can also lead to coma and death. [8]

That's a pretty graphic description of the disease, but is factually correct. JDRF (formerly the Juvenile Diabetes Research Foundation, now just JDRF) offers this description of type 1 diabetes:

Type 1 diabetes (T1D) is an autoimmune disease in which a person's pancreas stops producing insulin, a hormone that enables people to get energy from food. It occurs when the body's immune system attacks and destroys the insulin-producing cells in the pancreas, called beta cells. While its causes are not yet entirely understood, scientists believe that both genetic factors and environmental triggers are involved. Its onset has nothing to do with diet or lifestyle. There is nothing you can do to prevent T1D, and— at present—nothing you can do to get rid of it. [9]

Each of these descriptions of type 1 diabetes is a little different, but they share a number of facts in common:

- The pancreas stops producing insulin;
- Without adequate insulin, the body cannot normalize blood sugars;
- If blood sugars are not normalized, high blood sugar levels can result in a number of complications such as eye or kidney damage, increased risk for heart disease and, in extreme cases, coma and/or death;
- Taking insulin appropriately helps normalize blood sugar levels;
- There is nothing to be done to prevent type 1 diabetes, nor can you get rid of it.

Nothing you have done as a parent caused your child to get type 1 diabetes. Nothing!

Nothing your child has done, or not done, caused him or her to get type 1 diabetes. Nothing!

How is type 1 diabetes typically treated?

Your doctor and health care professional team have described a treatment for your child with type 1 diabetes, and the treatment has no doubt already begun. As a parent, you will want to work collaboratively with your health care team to design and carry out a treatment plan. We encourage you to learn as much as you can about treatment plans, as you serve as the primary advocate for your child.

As a parent, how do you know whether the treatment plan initially outlined by your child's physician child is the right or best one? There is no easy or single answer to this question. There are, however, some suggestions in the literature that may be useful to you as you consider your child's treatment plan.

The web site TeensHealth suggests a number of factors that must be addressed in a treatment plan for type 1 diabetes:

> A treatment plan, also called a diabetes management plan, helps people to manage their diabetes and stay healthy and active. Everyone's plan is different, based on a person's health needs and the suggestions of the diabetes health care team.
>
> - *Know your numbers*. The first thing to understand when it comes to treating diabetes is your blood

glucose level, which is the amount of glucose in the blood. To know blood glucose levels, a person with diabetes must check their glucose level several (number of times should be specified in the treatment plan) times each day.

- *Take Insulin every day.* People who have type 1 diabetes must take insulin as part of their treatment. Because their bodies can't make insulin anymore, they need to get the right amount to keep their blood sugar levels in a healthy range.
- *Eat a Healthy, Balanced Diet.* People with type 1 diabetes have to pay a little more attention to their meals and snacks than people who don't have diabetes. They need to eat a balanced, healthy diet and pay closer attention to what they eat and when they eat it.
- *Exercise Regularly.* Exercise is also an important part of diabetes treatment. Regular physical activity helps keep blood sugar levels in a healthy range. It also can reduce the risk of other health problems that people with diabetes may be more likely to get, like heart disease. [10]

WebMD offers an overview of type 1 diabetes treatment:

The goal of your child's treatment for type 1 diabetes is to always keep his or her blood sugar levels within a target range. A target range reduces the chance of diabetes complications. Daily diabetes care and regular medical checkups will help you and your child accomplish this goal.

Your child's daily care includes:

- Exercise. Experts recommend that teens and children (starting at age 6) do moderate to vigorous activity at least 1 hour every day.1
- Home blood sugar monitoring.
- Preparing and giving insulin injections.
- Living with an insulin pump.
- Counting carbohydrates.
- Dealing with low blood sugar levels.
- Preventing high blood sugar levels. [11]

And the Joslin Diabetes Center says this about treatment plans:

But when a treatment plan results in blood glucose levels that are normal or nearly so, a person's risk of developing complications drops dramatically. There are certain things that you need to do religiously in order to be healthy: Take insulin injections, follow a meal plan, and be physically active (physical activity can help the body better use insulin, so it can convert glucose into energy for cells). You'll have to monitor your blood glucose closely; regular testing will help determine how well the steps you're taking are working to keep blood glucose levels in a normal range

People with type 1 diabetes must take daily insulin injections, since they produce little or none on their own. Insulin is a vital hormone that helps the body convert food into energy. Without it, glucose builds up to intolerable levels in the bloodstream; untreated, patients die.

But in the early stages, shortly after diagnosis, many patients experience a "honeymoon period" during which the need for injected insulin is minimal; some people can actually maintain normal or near-normal blood glucose taking little or no insulin. This occurs because at this point in the disease's progression, a small percentage of the body's insulin-producing cells are still in operation. The disease may even appear to go away, since symptoms may emerge when the patient has an illness, then subside along with the illness as insulin needs decrease. But the process that has destroyed most of the insulin-producing cells will ultimately destroy the remaining cells. [12]

WebMD article describes some problems you may encounter, including:

- Changing appetite and "picky eating." A registered dietitian can help you develop a flexible meal plan to meet your child's appetite needs and allow for special events, such as parties and school activities. If you use rapid-acting insulin, you can give the insulin dose after a meal based on what your child ate. Some tips for mealtimes with young children include having alternative meal choices.
- Illness. Follow the sick-day guidelines that you and your child's doctor set up to prevent high blood sugar emergencies when your child is ill. Talk with the doctor before giving your child any nonprescription medicine.
- Exercise. If your child is not very active, limit his or her time playing video games, watching TV, or using the computer. Plan some activities to do along with your child, such as in-line skating or bicycling. Keep your child safe during exercise by:
- Checking his or her blood sugar levels before and after vigorous activity.
- Having a quick-sugar food on hand at all times.

- Giving the coach a copy of the symptoms of low blood sugar and instructions about what to do if it occurs. [13]

We encourage you to work closely with your health care team to design and implement a treatment plan that is right for your child. To get there, you need to ask questions until you get answers you can understand and are comfortable with. If you and your child (to the extent possible) can be active in the treatment plan process, chances are good the outcome for your child will be more positive.

To be honest: I'm scared!

Blood sugar levels, meters, shots, insulin, diet, exercise, hypoglycemia, complications, treatment plans, doctors, family: this is a whole lot to cope with, and I am scared to death about doing something wrong. This is my *child* after all, not some abstract idea. What do I do?

So far in this booklet, we've tried to help you understand something about diabetes as a disease, and a little about how the disease is treated. No doubt your doctor and healthcare team have given you a lot more information and guidance about how to be a parent of a child with diabetes. Even with all information about type 1 diabetes and your child, you are probably still experiencing a high level of anxiety about how best to support your child, both immediately and in the long run. Your concerns, your fears, are "normal." That doesn't necessarily make you feel better.

In the remainder of this booklet, we'd like to share with you 10 ideas you may find useful as you confront the emotional aspects of beginning to live with the diabetes that is now a part of your family. You probably noted that most of the material above deals with what might be called the medical aspects of dealing with diabetes. These medical considerations are, of course, of great importance to you and your child, and deserve your attention and involvement.

But managing your child's diabetes is not just a medical challenge; diabetes causes severe stresses and strains that tax the psychological and emotional strengths of all those involved. The ten ideas below are focused on these psychological and emotional issues that ultimately consume a substantial share of your time and effort in helping your child manage his or her diabetes. These ideas have emerged as a result of listening to scores of parents as they cope with diabetes in their families.

Ten things to know about the emotional and behavioral side of life with diabetes

1. Tough feelings are normal.

Shock, sadness, guilt, anger, fear and worry are a common reaction to getting the news that your child has diabetes. These feelings are a normal part of the grief and acceptance process. Does knowing that this is normal make it easier? Probably not, but it is important to recognize that you are not losing it, not going crazy, and certainly are not the only one who has ever had a difficult time with the transition of achild being diagnosed with type 1 diabetes.

Here's what some parents have felt when their child was diagnosed with diabetes:

> "On 23 April, 2004, our entire world changed. C was diagnosed with type 1 diabetes. It was the most traumatic thing that I have ever had to endure and I wouldn't wish it upon my worst enemy (not that I have any - I don't think).
>
> The first year was, and still is, a blur. I honestly don't know how we survived but somehow, we did. The strongest of all was C

- the one who had to endure countless blood glucose tests and endless needles. The one whose entire world had changed the most. SHE kept ME afloat. " [14]

"So, here it is....we ask the wrong question. When our children are diagnosed, when their blood sugars are off, when we're feeling overwhelmed and like this life is just too much for us, we ask the question "why". Why did God allow this to happen, why did it happen to us, why my child, why, why, why, why. It's always there, the question of why things are what they are. And we keep on asking it, no matter how many times we're denied the answer. And it finally occurred to me that there is no answer to that question." [15]

"Finding out your child has type 1 diabetes can be terrifying, and figuring out how to work diabetes care management into your life can be downright overwhelming. Right now you probably feel overwhelmed, confused and scared for your child. That's normal." [16]

"When a child is diagnosed with chronic illness, it's ordinary for parents to feel guilt and sadness. Anger is also common. You may

feel angry toward your partner, the world at
large or even, at times, toward your child.
These feelings are normal." [17]

2. You will get the hang of it.

It is often overwhelming to need to change so much and there is so much to learn: carbohydrate counting, handling hypoglycemia, blood glucose monitoring, meal planning, insulin regimens, and on and on. This is a lot to take in. Know that you will get more comfortable doing all that diabetes requires over the next few months.

A number of suggestions have been made for parents to cope with the first months after the diagnosis of type 1 diabetes in a child. Because diabetes is a highly personal illness, there cannot be a single "right way" to transition parental roles, but there are some ways that have been found to be effective in launching a parent and child's new life, and to help parents "get the hang" of managing these new lives. Here are some examples:

> The first step is to learn the skills needed to take care of the diabetes: how to draw up and inject insulin, how to measure blood glucose/sugar levels accurately, how to begin to plan meals and snacks. Older children will be part of this education program. For younger children, age-appropriate teaching will need to occur at a separate time. School-aged or older siblings and others intimately involved in the day-to-day care of the child such as babysitters or grandparents may also be involved in this program. In many centers, this education program takes place on an

out-patient basis, in some centers, even in the home.

For most families, it will take two or three days to learn the basics of diabetes care. If extra support is needed at the beginning, your diabetes team may arrange for home care to help you with injections and monitoring.

Knowledge is the basis of managing diabetes. Learn as much as you can about diabetes and how to manage it. This will help you feel more secure, and reduce your fears and concerns. The goal of diabetes management is to help children live long, healthy, productive lives, as much like any other child as possible. [18]

The message from this suggestion? The best way to "get the hang of it" is to learn all you can about diabetes; get started by learning the basics of diabetes care. In other words: be proactive! Don't try to hide from the reality of diabetes in your home.

Challenging – I'll bet it's challenging! So, what do we need to do? Great question! Let's talk about a few things that you will need to learn, such as:

- What happens in Jennifer's body when she eats or drinks
- How to monitor her blood glucose levels
- Signs and treatment of high and low blood glucose levels
- Jennifer's blood glucose target range (your doctor will tell you what blood glucose value is the best for your child. It may be a range of 80-140 mg/dl, for example)
- How to give insulin
- How to plan meals, snacks and count carbohydrates
- How to balance food, exercise, and insulin
- How to work with your diabetes health care team [19]

When you get into a tight place and everything goes against you, till it seems as though you could not hang on a minute longer, never give up then, for that is just the place and time that the tide will turn.

Harriet Beecher Stowe

3. Take it a day at a time.

Diabetes management can feel like a moving target. Hormones, your child's remaining insulin production, age and developmental issues all change over time. Therefore, what you and your child do to manage diabetes is going to change over time. Try to tackle the issues you are facing right now. Worrying about what problems your child may confront down the road (like in the teen years) when you are far from that now is not a good use of your energy today!

Taking things a day at a time seems like prudent advice, but what does it actually mean? Silverstein *et al* [23] published a statement called *Care of Children and Adolescents with Type 1 Diabetes,* in which they analyzed the position of the American Diabetes Association (ADA) on the topic of caring for children and adolescents with type 1 diabetes. The article provides an interesting perspective on the advice to "take things a day at a time," by indicating the developmental stages children and adolescents pass through, and the implications of those stages for priorities in diabetes care at each stage. In a sense, identifying developmental stages and coupling those stages with high-priority diabetes management tasks provides a clue as to what parents need to think about doing "a day at a time."

Following is a brief summary of the very important information provided by Silverstein et al. For each age group, the authors identify:

❖ The developmental task(s) a child undertakes in this age range;
➢ The diabetes management priority tasks that must be undertaken by the child and the parent in this age range; and
✓ The issues raised for the family by the developmental and diabetes management tasks to be undertaken in this age range.

Readers interested in learning more about these developmental and diabetes management tasks are urged to consult the Silverstein et al paper as listed in the Reference section of this booklet.

Development tasks, diabetes management priorities, and family issues

(From Silverstein et al [20])

Infancy (0-12 months

- ❖ Child's developmental tasks: Developing a trusting relationship/"bonding" with primary caregiver(s)
- ➤ Diabetes management priorities: Preventing and treating hypoglycemia; avoiding extreme fluctuations in blood glucose levels.
- ✓ Family issues: Coping with stress; sharing the "burden of care" to avoid parent burnout

Toddler (13–36 months)

- ❖ Child's developmental tasks: Developing a sense of mastery and autonomy
- ➤ Diabetes management priorities: Preventing and treating hypoglycemia; avoiding extreme fluctuations in blood glucose levels due to irregular food intake.
- ✓ Family issues: Establishing a schedule; managing the "picky eater;" setting limits and coping with toddler's lack of cooperation with regimen; and sharing the burden of care.

Pre-schooler and early elementary school age (3-7 years)

- ❖ Child's developmental tasks: Developing initiative in activities and confidence in self
- ➤ Diabetes management priorities: Preventing and treating hypoglycemia; unpredictable appetite and activity; positive reinforcement for cooperation with regimen; and trusting other caregivers with diabetes management.

✓ Family issues: Reassuring child that diabetes is no one's fault; and educating other caregivers about diabetes management.

Older elementary school-age (8–11 years)

❖ Child's developmental tasks: Developing skills in athletic, cognitive, artistic, social areas; and consolidating self-esteem with respect to the peer group.
➢ Diabetes management priorities: Making diabetes regimen flexible to allow for participation in school/peer activities; and child learning short- and long-term benefits of optimal control.
✓ Family issues: Maintaining parental involvement in insulin and blood glucose monitoring tasks while allowing for independent self-care for "special occasions;" and continue to educate school and other caregivers

Early adolescence (12–15 years)

❖ Child's developmental tasks: Managing body changes; and developing a strong sense of self-identity.
➢ Diabetes management priorities: Managing increased insulin requirements during puberty; Diabetes management and blood glucose control become more difficult; and there are weight and body image concerns.
✓ Family issues: Renegotiating parents and teen's roles in diabetes management to be acceptable to both; learning coping skills to enhance ability to self-manage; preventing and intervening with diabetes-related family conflict; and monitoring for signs of depression, learning disorders, risky behaviors.

Later adolescence (16–19 years)

- ❖ Child's developmental tasks: Establishing a sense of identity after high school (decision about location, social issues, work, education).
- ➢ Diabetes management priorities: Begin discussion of transition to a new diabetes team Integrating diabetes into new lifestyle.
- ✓ Family issues: Supporting the transition to independence; learning coping skills to enhance ability to self-manage; preventing and intervening with diabetes-related family conflict; and monitoring for signs of depression, eating disorders, risky behaviors. [20]

Parents are reminded that each child is different, and may not "align" exactly to these developmental tasks during the age range suggested. Perhaps the most important part of the paper is the identification of the diabetes management priorities. These priorities enable parents to prepare themselves for the next steps in their child's diabetes requirements.

4. **Work as a team in managing your child's diabetes**

You, your child, and your healthcare professionals need to all be on the same team in managing diabetes. Work with your child to think about "What now?" when learning how to make decisions about diabetes. Sometimes we do not know why wacky blood sugars happen, but it is important to be able to problem solve what to do next. Asking good questions is your most powerful tool! (What do you think would happen if...?) Make decisions together. Remember that success is the best teacher – focus on what you and your child are doing well.

The Team: Who should be on it?

The National Diabetes Education Program suggests the following for members of the diabetes healthcare team:

> Ideally, diabetes care for youth with diabetes should be provided by a team that can deal with the special medical, educational, nutritional, and behavioral issues associated with children and teens. The team usually consists of a physician, diabetes educator, dietitian, social worker or psychologist, along with the patient and family. [21]

The American Diabetes Association offers this advice:

Whether the initial care and education is given as an inpatient or an outpatient and whether this care is provided by a pediatric endocrinologist/diabetes team, an internist endocrinologist, or the child's primary care provider will depend on the age of the child, the ability to provide outpatient education, the clinical severity of the child at presentation, and the geographic proximity of the patient to a tertiary care center. Ideally, every child newly diagnosed with type 1 diabetes should be evaluated by a diabetes team consisting of a pediatric endocrinologist, a nurse educator, a dietitian, and a mental health professional qualified to provide up-to-date pediatric-specific education and support. Such systems of care, unfortunately, are not always available. In the future, greater use of telemedicine may allow the expertise of established pediatric centers to improve the care of children in remote areas. [22]

The Lehigh Valley Health Network identifies and describes members of a comprehensive type 1 diabetes care team:

Endocrinologist: An endocrinologist is a doctor who has special education in diabetes and related hormone disorders. Your endocrinologist may occasionally refer you to an eye doctor, foot doctor, heart doctor or other specialist. Each time you see one of these other health care providers, be sure the test results and other information are sent to your endocrinologist so he or she can stay up-to-date when coordinating your care.

Certified diabetes nurse educator: The nurse educator has special education in treating and caring for people with diabetes and will provide you with information about diabetes and teach you practical aspects of daily self-care. You'll receive instruction in everything from giving yourself insulin shots and checking your blood sugar to dealing with the symptoms of low blood sugar or insulin reactions.

Primary care physician: You will work closely with your primary care physician for regular checkups, test referrals and general medical care. Your primary care physician is a good resource for questions you may have about any symptoms that concern you, for referrals to specialists or for more information about diabetes.

Eye doctor: Diabetes can affect the blood vessels in the eyes and lead to blindness. Unfortunately, once the symptoms are apparent, the damage usually is irreversible. For this reason, the American Diabetes Association recommends that people with diabetes see their eye doctor – either an ophthalmologist or optometrist – at least once a year for preventive care. Choose an eye doctor with experience in identifying and treating diabetic eye disease.

Podiatrist: Uncontrolled diabetes may lead to poor blood flow, sores and infections in the feet and lower legs. A podiatrist specializes in these areas of the body and can identify potential problems before they become more serious.

Dentist: Because of the increased risks for gum disease and oral infections that come with diabetes, plan to see your dentist twice a year for regular visits. Be sure your dentist knows you have diabetes.

Registered dietitian: A registered dietitian works with you to determine an appropriate meal plan for you, based on your weight goals, the medications you take and other factors. Even if you have had diabetes for a while, consider talking with a registered dietitian. As you age, your nutritional needs can change.

Social worker/psychologist/psychiatrist/marriage

and family therapist: Managing a chronic illness involves many physical, emotional and economic challenges – not just for the person with diabetes, but also for your family. These professionals can help you and your family learn how to cope with the emotional issues and stress of living with diabetes. [23]

We add to these suggestions: ***Parents must be considered critical members of the health care team.*** Here is why:

The patient -- or for kids with diabetes, the parents -- are in charge of their diabetes care. As parents, we are the best advocates for our children. We see our kids everyday, we know how their bodies react to the stresses of school, sports, and everything else that is a part of their lives. Since we're in charge, the choices of which meter to use, whether to use pump therapy and -- if so -- which pump to use, when we'll eat, and everything else related to our care are ours to make. The members of the diabetes team provide guidance based on current medical science, advise us on therapy options, and help us learn how to live our lives as if we didn't have diabetes, to the extent that that is possible. The diabetes team is like the coaching staff of a sporting team, and we are like the players. The coaching staff helps us

learn the game, but the game is ours to play
and ours to win. [24]

Who else might you consider part of your team?

You may want to use the technologies available to you to
"add" members to your team: other parents of kids with
type 1 diabetes; bloggers who provide useful information;
online diabetes communities that connect you with a
significant number of people and ideas.

With your computer and an Internet connection, or with your
tablet or smartphone, the diabetes world opens to you. You
will need to roam around in this online community a bit, to
get a sense of who and what is out there, but you will no
doubt soon find the sites that best suit your needs.

To get you started, here are some Internet sites you
may wish to explore:

- Diabetes Mine: "A gold mine of straight talk and
  encouragement."
  http://www.diabetesmine.com/
- tuDiabetes.org: "A community of people touched by
  diabetes."
  http://www.tudiabetes.org/
- diaTribe: "Research and product news for people
  with diabetes."
  http://diatribe.us/
- Behavioral Diabetes Institute: "Tools to face the
  psychological demands of diabetes"
  www.behavioraldiabetes.org

- Children with diabetes: "The online community for kids, families and adults with diabetes"
  http://www.childrenwithdiabetes.com/
- Diabetes Daily
  http://www.diabetesdaily.com/
- Parenting diabetes kids
  http://www.parentingdiabetickids.com/
- Sixuntilme: "Diabetes doesn't define me, but it helps explain me."
  http://sixuntilme.com/wp/
- Diabetic Connect
  http://www.diabeticconnect.com/
- dLife: "It's your diabetes life!"
  http://www.dlife.com/
- Taking Control of Your Diabetes (TCOYD): "Educating and Empowering the Diabetes Community since 1995."
  http://tcoyd.org/
- Diabetes Forum
  http://www.diabetesforum.com/forum.php
- International Diabetes Federation, Diabetes Online Community: "Diabetes: Protect our Future."
  http://www.idf.org/worlddiabetesday/toolkit/pwd/diabetes-online-community

And on-and-on: There are so much out there on the Internet that make it possible for you to find supporters, colleagues, experts, people who have been where you are. It may be worth your time to find some people from the diabetes online community to "join" your team.

5. Help you child learn to do the "tasks" of diabetes him or herself as soon as feasible.

Research has shown that children who learn how to control their own blood glucose grow up to achieve better control and better emotional health. Obviously, what tasks your child will be able to do successfully will depend a lot on his or her age, maturity, and abilities. Work to turn over diabetes tasks as your child develops.

The point is well-taken, but oh how difficult this is for a parent, particularly the parent of a very young child newly diagnosed with type 1 diabetes. Parents, this is going to be tough on you, but it is necessary.

JDRF put the issue this way:

> One of your most important jobs as the parent of a child with T1D is to supervise, encourage, and foster the independence your child needs to successfully manage T1D. Try to avoid being overprotective.

> Overly protective parents undermine a child's self-esteem. Instead of developing a feeling of mastery over his or her environment, the child may develop a "sickly" self-image, use T1D to exert control, use low blood sugar as a means to avoid unpleasant activities, or let high blood sugar develop to a point of crisis.

> Self-care is the key to the development of a
> child's independence and self-esteem. This
> point cannot be overstated: You must get
> your child involved in self-care as soon as he
> or she is able to master self-management
> tasks and is emotionally ready. At the same
> time, supervision by caregivers must
> continue. [25]

Rather blunt, but also quite to the point: the child with type
1 diabetes who has a good handle on the tasks needed to live
with diabetes will be well-served for a lifetime with diabetes.

Even parents who acknowledge the importance of promoting
independence in diabetes self-management may not find it
easy to do so.

> When and how to transfer responsibility for
> diabetes management from the parent to
> the child or adolescent is an important issue
> to consider. From a very young age, children
> can be encouraged to participate in
> developmentally appropriate diabetes tasks
> under the gentle guidance and watchful eyes
> of their parents. However, pushing
> youngsters too hard to autonomy may lead
> to serious problems. Adolescents who
> assume diabetes responsibilities too soon
> face an increased risk of problems with
> treatment adherence, poor metabolic
> control and preventable hospitalizations.

> Total autonomy with diabetes self-
> management is not a reasonable goal for
> adolescents. [26]

What makes the tasks of diabetes self-management difficult for children and adolescents? The answer is, regrettably, many things.

- Both parents and child experience highly-charged emotions following diagnosis, and often for some time beyond that. These emotions may make it very difficult for teaching and learning of basic diabetes management skills to occur.

> The diagnosis of type 1 diabetes represents a crisis for children and parents. Family members often experience the classic stages of grief as they begin to grapple with the lifelong nature of diabetes and its potential consequences. In the first few months, it is common for children and adolescents to feel sad, lonely, anxious and irritable. Outbursts of temper, pessimism about the future, and refusal to take insulin or go to school are less common responses and more cause for concern. Parents, especially mothers, also report feelings of depression and anxiety, which may be precipitated by guilt or worry

about the child's future. These negative reactions in youngsters and their parents seem to be normative responses, and they tend to subside during the first year. When adjustment problems persist, however, there is greater risk for later problems with psychosocial adjustment and metabolic control. [27]

- Children pass through developmental stages in different ways. The developmental stage of the child plays a role in the child's willingness and/or ability to learn and exercise diabetes self-management strategies.

A not to be overlooked reality: managing diabetes is a complex task, so it is not so easy to learn all that is required. A fascinating paper by Ronald Coffen [28] argues that there are no fewer than 600 discrete tasks in the management of diabetes.

At first glance, one might assume that these high stakes would motivate youth with diabetes to take good care of themselves. Why, then, might that not be what is found? Why do youth struggle to follow the regimen designed for their own health? It is the premise here that it is due, in part, to the

magnitude of what these youth are required
to remember to do daily, even hourly, with
no "vacation." [29]

So how do parents go about transferring responsibility of the child's management of diabetes from the parent to the child? Slowly and carefully, with love and support. Here are some ideas you may find useful:

CVS offers some general suggestions for thinking
about the responsibilities of your child, at different
ages, for managing his or her diabetes:

Infants and Toddlers
Children under the age of two are too young to
understand what's going on. Stay calm and try to test
blood and inject insulin quickly. Comfort and
reassure your child afterward.

Preschool Children
Explain diabetes-related terms and what you are
doing to treat the disease, simply and often. Make
sure your child understands they did not do anything
to cause diabetes and the steps you take allow them
to control it. Reiterate that controlling diabetes
allows them to do what they love doing. This
reassurance should be repeated beyond your child's
preschool years.

Children 5-12 Years Old

Slowly let your child take on more diabetes-related tasks such as meal planning and doing blood sugar checks, but stay involved. Use your child's maturity, skills, readiness, and interest to help you determine how much they are ready for and when. Also, answer any questions your child has and make sure they can talk comfortably about the disease. This will help their peers feel comfortable with diabetes too.

Teenagers

The teenage years can be a time of rebellion and experimentation. Puberty brings growth spurts and body changes, making glucose control more difficult. This may lead to poor diabetes management. Teens usually do not consider the consequences of skipping tests and injections. They may not understand or worry about the long-term implications of poor glucose control and the dangers that diabetes carries.

Help your teenager through this time by being honest, sensitive, and supportive. Teach teens the facts about diabetes and how the choices they make will affect them. Get help from teachers or counselors if necessary. Don't forget, Try to anticipate teenage temptations such as alcohol and give your teenager the tools they need to address these temptations without creating diabetic disasters. [30]

An interesting research study was undertaken in which a child with type 1 diabetes, and one of his or her parents, were paired together and interviewed about diabetes self-management. The children were old enough to understand and answer the interview questions, so obviously very young children were not included in the study.

As there were only 22 children involved, generalizing too much from this study should be avoided, yet the results were interesting.

> Self-management of type I diabetes is key to good physical and psychosocial outcomes of the disease, yet little is known about how youth and their parents share responsibility for illness management. This study describes the division of labor between youth and their parents, self-management conflict, and three patterns of self-management in youth across four developmental stages: preadolescence, early adolescence, mid-adolescence, and late adolescence.

> Results (of the study) indicated that parents of preadolescents (8–11 years) performed much of their children's diabetes care. Dyads (A child plus his/her parent) reported some conflicts, particularly over food, amount of bolus, and blood glucose testing. The dyads demonstrated a self-management pattern that we identified as parent-dominant.

Most early adolescents (11–15 years) performed much of their own daily care, but parents actively participated in their self-management and oversaw it. The majority of dyads reported conflict over food and blood glucose testing. Most early adolescents demonstrated a transitional self-management pattern whereby they managed their own daily care, with varying amounts of parental oversight. In mid-adolescence (15–17 years), youth managed nearly all of their diabetes care; however, some dyads reported that parental oversight of illness care was still considerable.

Exercise was conflictual for the majority of these dyads. Over half of the youth and, by late adolescence (17–19 years), all youth demonstrated a pattern of adolescent-dominant self-management. In adolescent-dominant self-management, youth independently managed their diabetes. Half of the dyads reported that there were sometimes conflicts over food and blood glucose testing. more targeted assistance to youth with diabetes and to their parents.[31]

Finally, a few words about the special case of teenagers with type 1 diabetes. JDRF offers these observations:

If your child is a teenager: Understanding and recognizing the limits of your control are key elements in helping your teenager with T1D work through the challenges of adolescence. Three areas of special importance are:

- o Understand the Need for Spontaneity. Teens want to be spontaneous—to be able to do things, eat things, try things. T1D requires the opposite. A teen with T1D must realize that freedom only comes with knowledge and responsibility. Only by fully understanding and controlling his or her diabetes can a teen achieve the flexibility he or she craves
- o Understand the Need for Control. Teens want to be masters of their own lives. They want to define their own identities. To accomplish these objectives, they have to keep testing their limits. You can help show how they can use the discipline and control of diabetes care to gain strength and mastery in other parts of their lives.
- o Recognize the Limits of Your Control. Be realistic. Accept the fact that you can't watch over your teen every minute of the day. You, too, have to learn that it's your child's T1D, not yours.

By no means do these suggestions mean you should turn your back on your teen and allow him or her to self-destruct. You can talk with your teen about the choices he or she is making. Talk about grown-up matters, like career, marriage, and alcohol. Talking with your teenager shows you think of him or her as an adult and helps keep the lines of communication open during this difficult period. [32]

6.   As a parent, you are the assistant coach and the cheerleader, not the diabetes police.

Your child needs to know that, while he or she will bear ultimate responsibility for diabetes management, he/she is not alone in diabetes management. You are watching out and encouraging, are there for guidance, and will follow through with known consequences for lapses in responsibility. When you see blood glucose numbers, try not to use words like "good" and "bad", or make comments or faces. Try to treat these numbers as pieces of information that will help you make better decisions (at times this may require your best poker face).

Diabetes police is an often-used term in the diabetes community. For the most part, the connotation is negative, at least in the eyes of the person with diabetes. Just who is the diabetes police?

> They're here, they're there, they're everywhere! It's the Diabetes Police—your family, friends and others who criticize your diabetes behaviors. They disapprove of your food choices, point out your weight gain, accuse you of skipping your medication and nag you to exercise more. These well-meaning individuals care about you, but they

make life with diabetes more difficult and can create tension in a relationship. [33]

So the diabetes police force is comprised of family, friends, and others you come in contact with. And the force means well!

> If it hasn't happened yet, it will soon. You'll reach for a treat and a close friend, family member, or even a near-stranger who knows you have diabetes will ask: "Should you be eating that?"

> You've just been pulled over by a member of the "diabetes police"—well-meaning citizens concerned about your ability to manage blood sugar on your own. They probably want to help, but constant nagging about every bit of food you put in your mouth "tends to just work against people with diabetes instead of for them," says Constance Brown-Riggs, a nutritionist and certified diabetes educator in Massapequa, N.Y. [34]

As a parent, how do you best help your child deal with the inevitable diabetes police in his or her life? First and foremost, try not to enlist in the diabetes police force yourself. Sounds easy enough, but sometimes it's difficult not acting like a member of the diabetes police. There will be many moments in your relationship with your child when, in the immortal words of Archie Bunker, you will need to "stifle yourself."

Be sensitive to what your child thinks the diabetes police say or do to them. Listen to these things even if you want to protest that "you don't do those things." You may not, but others might.

The Behavioral Diabetes Institute (BDI) distributes a small brochure called a diabetes etiquette care for parents, in which teens indicate what they would like their parents to know. The main points stressed in the brochure are:

- o Stop trying to scare me with diabetes statistics.
- o When my blood sugars are high, don't assume I've done something stupid (although I may have).
- o Please acknowledge when I'm doing something right, not just when I've messed up.
- o Don't always be in my face about diabetes, but don't leave me completely alone with it either.
- o Make the effort to understand diabetes from my point of view.
- o Don't tell everyone about my diabetes, especially during the first minute you meet them.
- o Recognize that I am never going to be perfect with my diabetes care, no matter how much you want this.
- o Don't limit my activities based on diabetes.
- o Don't be the food police. [35]

If you were able to do (or not do) these things, you would not hold membership in the diabetes police, which would be a very good thing!

Is there anything you as a parent can do to reduce the diabetes police behavior on the part of other family members, friends, or people off the street? Yes. The OneTouch web site offers suggestions:

- o The people closest to you need to learn about diabetes. Diabetes is a self-managed disease and it is essential that you learn all you can about how to deal with it.
- o You need to let your family and friends know what you expect of them. As you begin to get a handle on the disease, you need to let the people closest to you know what you want from them.
- o The better job [your child] does of controlling his/her blood sugar levels, the less effect diabetes will have on your family and friends. [36]

7. Be prepared for some insensitive and often ignorant comments from others about the diabetes in your family.

When people learn about your child's diagnosis, you may hear ignorant responses that reflect myths about diabetes, outdated knowledge, insensitive personal stories, and unsolicited advice. In time, it is possible you can help your friends and family better understand diabetes, and its role in your household. In time, but probably not right away. You will need to endure the unfortunate comments from friends and family, even if those comments are well-intentioned.

So why do people stress and embarrass you with questions that are simply off-the-wall, and my be highly disturbing to your child? There's no simple answer to this question, but a generous way of excusing such unfortunate comments is that family and friends simply do not know enough, or know the right stuff, about diabetes. And it is highly likely that many of the people with whom you associate are victims of myths about diabetes.

To help you understand where some of your friends and colleagues are coming from, it may benefit you to know about some of the common myths circulating about the nature of diabetes, based on which some people form very ill-informed ideas and opinions about the disease, which often translates into inappropriate question or comments coming to you.

Following are some of the myths "out there" about diabetes that may be contributing to the kinds of verbal abuse you and your family get about your child and diabetes:

These 10 myths were compiled by Diabetes.co.uk

- Myth #1: People with diabetes can't eat sugar
- Myth #2: Type 2 diabetes is mild
- Myth #3: Type 2 diabetes only affects fat people
- Myth #4: People with diabetes should only eat diabetic food
- Myth #5: People with diabetes go blind and lose their legs
- Myth #6: People with diabetes are dangerous drivers
- Myth #7: People with diabetes shouldn't play sport
- Myth #8: People with diabetes can't do many jobs
- Myth #9: People with diabetes are more likely to be ill
- Myth #10: Diabetes is contagious [37]

The American Diabetes Association also assembled a list of diabetes myths that may inform people about diabetes, which in term may be reflected in the questions or comments of friends, family, and acquaintances:

- Myth: Diabetes is not that serious of a disease.
- Myth: If you are overweight or obese, you will eventually develop type 2 diabetes.
- Myth: Eating too much sugar causes diabetes.
- Myth: People with diabetes should eat special diabetic foods.

- Myth: If you have diabetes, you should only eat small amounts of starchy foods, such as bread, potatoes and pasta.
- Myth: People with diabetes can't eat sweets or chocolate.
- Myth: You can catch diabetes from someone else.
- Myth: People with diabetes are more likely to get colds and other illnesses.
- Myth: If you have type 2 diabetes and your doctor says you need to start using insulin, it means you're failing to take care of your diabetes properly.
- Myth: Fruit is a healthy food. Therefore, it is ok to eat as much of it as you wish. [38]

Finally, here are some myths about type 1 diabetes, from JDRF:

> We all know a diagnosis of type 1 diabetes (T1D) is hard on families as they learn to cope with a number of changes in their daily life. While people care, it is all too common for them to ask questions that reflect a lack of knowledge about T1D, such as, "When will she outgrow it?" It can be frustrating to explain the battle that all families face every hour of every day, and that can be compounded by having to deal with people's common misunderstandings and misperceptions, including the widely-held belief that T1D is not a serious disease. Here are some of those myths:

- Myth: Taking insulin cures diabetes.
- Myth: Diabetes is caused by obesity, or eating too much sugar.
- Myth: With strict adherence to a specific diet and exercise plan, and multiple insulin injections each day based on careful monitoring of blood sugar levels, a person with T1D can easily gain tight control over his or her blood sugar levels.
- Myth: People with diabetes should never eat sweets.
- Myth: People with diabetes can't participate in athletics.
- Myth: Only kids get type 1 diabetes.
- Myth: Kids don't get type 2 diabetes.
- Myth: Women with diabetes shouldn't get pregnant.
- Myth: No matter what you do, a person with diabetes for years will eventually get complications. [39]

With this long list of myths about diabetes out there, is it any wonder that many people are misinformed about the nature of diabetes, and thus ask questions or make comments that not at all helpful to either children with diabetes or their parents? To the extent you can enlighten others about the truths of diabetes, the sooner the inappropriate questions may stop.

8.   You (the parent) matter too!

Your own self-care is critical for being able to maintain the emotional and physical strength for facing the on-going daily challenges with your child's diabetes. Although it is very hard to make yourself a priority during this stressful time following the diagnosis of diabetes, your own exercise, diabetes-free time (no matter how small), as well as time with your spouse, other children and family can help you "refuel". And you need to be re-fueled at regular intervals.

Is caregiver stress actually an issue?

In a word: Yes. If you are experiencing a great deal of stress since you child was diagnosed with type 1 diabetes, you would be wise to acknowledge the stress to yourself and others.

> Researchers have identified something called "Caregiver Stress Syndrome" which is characterized by grief, anxiety and feelings of helplessness. People with Caregiver Stress Syndrome may also experience insomnia (rates as high as 86%) and fatigue related to taking care of an ill loved one. These symptoms result from both acute, or immediate, stress such as a serious flare up in symptoms requiring hospitalization and chronic, long term, stress from managing

day-to-day tasks like taking medications or calling doctor's offices for test results. [40]

Consider this observation:

Caregiving Can Damage the Health of the Caregiver

Caregiving can be very damaging on the health of the caregiver. According to a study published in 1999 in the Journal of the American Medical Association researchers Richard Schulz and Scott Beach from University of Pittsburgh reported that elderly caregivers are at a 63 percent higher risk of mortality than noncaregivers in the same age group.

They found that the physical symptoms of caregiver stress are a result of a prolonged and elevated level of stress hormones circulating in the body. Researchers likened exhausted caregivers' stress hormone levels to those suffering from post traumatic stress disorder.

Additionally, the chronic stress of caring for someone can lead to high blood pressure, diabetes and a compromised immune system. [41]

Caregiver burn-out

When a child has diabetes, it can be seem
like an all-consuming, never-ending string of
tasks that gradually take over your entire life.
When you begin to feel this way, you are
either close to or in what is commonly called
caregiver burnout. This is a term that
describes many people who are caring for a
person with a demanding chronic condition
like diabetes. It is not unique to diabetes, but
is very common among parents of children
with type 1 diabetes. [42]

As a parent, you will find it difficult, if not impossible, to
provide the kind of care your child with type 1 diabetes
requires, if you are simply not up to the task. The
characteristics of diabetes listed above (all-consuming,
never-ending string of tasks) apply to the caregiver as well as
the person with diabetes.

Gary Gilles, the author of the web site article cited above,
suggests there are three primary indicators that your own
capacity as a caregiver is growing thin:

1. Negative feelings toward your child: When you feel
    resentment toward your child for the needs they
    have pertaining to diabetes, you know that you are
    close to caregiver burnout.
2. Social isolation: There are times when the care that
    you provide for your child can seem to crowd out
    needed time with others. A feeling of social isolation

can creep in where you begin to feel very alone in this journey of parenting and diabetes.

3. Poor self-care: some parents who struggle with feeling worthy to have needs use their child with diabetes to justify ignoring their own. Not only does this potentially put your health and important relationships at risk but it also sends the wrong message to your child about responsible self-care. [43]

What can I do as a parent to keep myself healthy while caring for my child with type 1 diabetes?

There is no single right answer to this question, but there are a lot of ideas that have been expressed for how you might keep yourself fit while helping to manage your child's diabetes. Following are a few strategies that have been suggested:

WebMD offers the following tips:

What Can I Do to Reduce Caregiver Stress in My Life?

- Keep a positive attitude. Believe in yourself.
- Accept that there are events you cannot control.
- Be assertive instead of aggressive. "Assert" your feelings, opinions, or beliefs instead of becoming angry, combative, or passive.
- Learn to relax.
- Exercise regularly. Your body can fight stress better when it is fit.
- Stop smoking.

- Limit yourself to moderate alcohol and caffeine intake.
- Set realistic goals and expectations.
- Get enough rest and sleep. Your body needs time to recover from stressful events.
- Don't rely on alcohol or drugs to reduce stress.
- Learn to use stress management techniques and coping mechanisms, such as deep breathing or guided imagery. [44]

The United States Department of Health and Human Services offers these tips:
When it comes to their health, caregivers are less likely than their peers to take steps
to prevent or control chronic disease. Taking care of your own health will help you to better care for your loved one longer.

- Be wise – immunize.
  - Influenza (flu) vaccine: The CDC recommends that caregivers of the elderly (we add and children with diabetes) get one each year.
  - Pneumococcal vaccination: For most caregivers, one will last a lifetime.
  - Tetanus booster: Get one every ten years.
- Don't neglect your health.
  - Get a yearly check-up and the recommended cancer screenings (mammogram, cervical screening, etc.).

- o Tell your doctor that you are a caregiver.
- o Tell your doctor if you feel depressed or nervous.
- o Take some time each day to do something for yourself. Read, listen to music, telephone friends, or exercise.
- o Eat healthy foods and do not skip meals.
- o Find caregiver resources in your area early. You may not need their information or services now, but you will have them, when you need them.
- o Don't be afraid to ask for help. And don't do it all yourself. Use your family, friends, or neighbors for support. Family may help share caregiving tasks. Friends and neighbors may help with other chores. [45]

Parents Magazine offered this suggestion:

Handling chronic illness is about learning to live in balance," says Rosalind Dorlen, Psy.D., a psychotherapist with Overlook Hospital, in Summit, New Jersey, who specializes in treating the depression and anxiety that often accompany long-term health problems. "You can't dwell on questions like, 'Why is this happening to me?' or 'What if it gets worse?' But you do have to be constantly conscious of your health status, and take the time to rest, exercise, and have fun. It's important to focus on feeling well and to

maintain a positive outlook." And many
parents have learned to do just that. [46]

9. You (and your child) don't have to be perfect to live a long, happy, and healthy life with diabetes.

Perfect diabetes management is neither possible nor necessary for good health. In fact, striving for perfection is a set up for discouragement and feelings of burn out. Instead, work towards a goal of "healthy good enough". This goal is ambitious yet realistic, takes into account individual and family needs, is flexible, and changes over time as the needs change. Be encouraged! There is good evidence that with good (not perfect) care, your child can live a healthy life with diabetes.

The literature is filled with exhortations to people with diabetes, and parents of children with diabetes, not to demand or expect perfection in diabetes management. Here are several examples of what has been said on the topic:

> "Expecting 100 percent can be a set up for a letdown. Behind the science and technology of healthcare are humans. And humans aren't perfect. Healthcare professionals aren't always so responsive. Delays are going to happen, along with the restrictions and inconveniences of managed care.
>
> And then there are family members, who aren't always so supportive, because they aren't able to or don't know how to, or just won't. And you're human too. With good

days and bad days, good intentions, and your own limitations.

So, given that we are dealing with imperfect beings, what if, instead of expecting perfection, you expected imperfection? What if you started to ask yourself what parts of your life need to be functioning at 100 percent, and where you might begin to loosen up on your expectations? Averaging out your expectations to, let's say, around 80 percent? This would mean allowing for the human factor in yourself and others. It might also mean a whole lot less disappointment. Not to mention a whole lot less stress." [47]

Perfectionism. Something else that fosters the development of diabetes burnout, and consequently serves as a sign that burnout is on the horizon, is when parents have to have perfection. This usually plays out by aiming for blood glucose levels that are always in a very tight range, and constantly searching for the reasons for "bad" blood glucose levels.

Don't get us wrong: We are advocates of intensive diabetes management and help families find ways to carry out the behaviors needed to achieve the safest and healthiest control of diabetes possible. However, aiming for perfection typically leads to frustration, disappointment, and ultimately diabetes burnout.

The problem with aiming for perfection is that so many things go into achieving optimal control, and you can't control all of them. Diabetes management is not always predictable. The cause for a high blood glucose level today may not be the same cause of the high blood glucose level tomorrow. When you set out to have all perfect blood glucose levels or that perfect A1C level, you can set yourself up for feeling like a failure. Anything that falls short of perfect, even if it is the best you and your family can do at that time, may cause guilt and blame and diabetes burnout. [48]

There is just no place for perfectionism in diabetes management (or in any area of life, actually). It just leads to beating yourself up and sapping your self-confidence. And then, why keep trying if you "just can't do it," as Lia said?

But perfectionism is hard to let go. In most cases, we learned it as young children. You have to please the adults in your life, or you'll get in trouble. To please them you have to be perfect. It's not easy to unlearn that lesson. If you are inclined to perfectionism, you might want to get some help. [49]

Many people don't realize that keeping blood glucose levels "normal" is an impossible goal. Even if you are somehow able to eat the same food at the same time every day and do the same exercise for the same length of time at the same hour every day--all while taking the same amount of insulin or other medication—your blood glucose is going to fluctuate.

Blood glucose levels can be affected by hormones, stress levels, weather, emotional issues and a host of other factors we don't even know about. No matter how careful you are, your body will not always respond the way you expect it to. And that's okay.

Try not to despair. Or feel "less than," guilty, like a failure or aggravated by your situation. The fact is, there's no such thing as a "perfect" person with diabetes or "perfect" control. As long as you take your medication or insulin as directed, follow your food plan to the best of your ability and adhere to your medical team's advice regarding exercise, you need not be overly concerned about small fluctuations in your blood sugar; these are just part of managing diabetes.

It's easy to be self-critical or to become disheartened when it seems like nothing works. But remember, things are working: it's completely normal to experience variations in blood sugar levels. If, however, you're having repeat episodes of unusually high or low blood sugar, talk to your medical team. You may be developing an infection or experiencing hormonal or other changes that need attention.

The bottom line is control your diabetes as best you can, but never let it control you. [50]

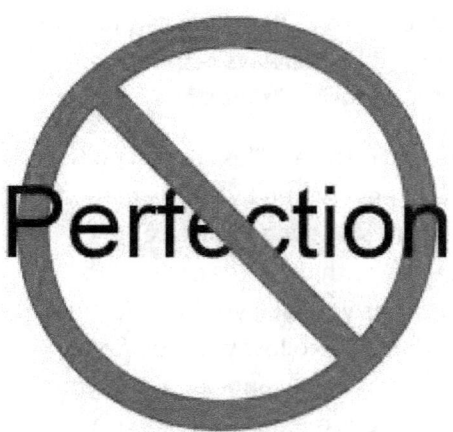

Retrieved from: http://ripplerevolution.com/saynotoperfection/

10. Your child can live a long and healthy life with diabetes!

While you deal with the immediate challenges of helping your child (and your family) adjust to the presence of type 1 diabetes in the household, you probably think a bit about the long-term implications for your child with diabetes. *Life expectancy* with diabetes inevitably raises its head as an issue. What do we know about this topic? Briefly:

> Life expectancy at birth for someone diagnosed with type 1 diabetes between 1965 and 1980 was estimated to be 68.8 years compared to 72.4 years for the general population. But, for someone diagnosed with type 1 diabetes between 1950 and 1964 the estimated life expectancy at birth was just 53.4 years.

> The gap between life expectancy for people with type 1 diabetes (diagnosed between 1965 and 1980) and the general U.S. population is now just four years, according to the study. [51]

And:

> The life expectancy of people diagnosed with type 1 diabetes dramatically increased during the course of a 30-year, long-term prospective study, according to researchers at the University of Pittsburgh whose

findings currently appear online in the journal Diabetes.

The life expectancy for participants diagnosed with type 1 diabetes between 1965 and 1980 was 68.8 years – a 15-year improvement, compared to those diagnosed between 1950 and 1964, according to the study. Meanwhile, the life expectancy of the general U.S. population increased less than one year during the same time period. [52]

And:

The largest and most accurate assessment of contemporary life expectancy in people with type 1 diabetes to date shows they are almost certainly living much longer than they have historically.

The new analysis shows, for example, that those with type 1 diabetes are living around 11 to 14 years less, on average, at the age of 20 to 24 years than those in the general population; this figure drops to 5 to 7 years less at age 65 to 69. In the past, life expectancy has differed by as much as 27 years between those with type 1 diabetes and the general population, she pointed out. [53]

The trend is clear: people with diabetes are living longer than ever before. With these extended years comes extended medical requirements and expenses, hopes and fears. But for a parent at the time of seeing his or her child diagnosed with type 1 diabetes, comfort can be taken that this child will live a long life and, with the help of family and friends, a happy life.

Summing up

In this e-booklet, we have acknowledged how shocking and upsetting it can be for a parent to learn his or her child has type 1 diabetes. We very briefly described the nature of type 1 diabetes, and some of the ways the disease is treated.

Recognizing the many, if not most, parents struggle with how to assimilate type 1 diabetes into the life of their child and the entire family. The heart of this e-booklet is the ten ideas or tips we make to parents trying to figure out what to do next to help their child cope with, and even thrive with, type 1 diabetes. The ten tips include:

- Idea 1: Tough feelings are normal.
- Idea 2: You will get the hang of it.
- Idea 3: Take it a day at a time.
- Idea 4: Work as a team in managing diabetes.
- Idea 5: Help your child learn to do the tasks of diabetes him/herself as soon as feasible.
- Idea 6: You are the assistant coach and the cheerleader, not the diabetes police.
- Idea 7: Be prepared for some insensitive and often ignorant comments from others about the diabetes in your family.
- Idea 8: You (the parent) matter too!
- Idea 9: You (and your child) don't have to perfect to live a long, healthy and happy life with diabetes.
- Idea 10: The life expectancy of a young person today, diagnosed with type 1 diabetes, is less than a person without diabetes, but the gap is narrowing.

While these ideas will not make your child's type 1 diabetes go away, the ideas may be useful to you in developing a positive approach to management of your child's diabetes. With "good enough" management, you and your entire family can live the new diabetes life with energy and optimism!

We at Dynamic Diabetes Solutions extend to you our continuing support and encouragement. Thank you for reading this e-booklet.

References

Note: Full bibliographic citations are not provided for each of the sources cited in this document. Rather, each reference is identified only by its Internet address (URL) and title of the site from which information or a quote was obtained. The purpose of the reference list is to introduce readers to a wide range of resources available to them on the Internet, and to acknowledge the source of content included in this document.

Web sites come and go, change, and update on a regular basis. Therefore, we cannot guarantee that each URL listed below is still live or active. All were active at the time this e-booklet was written, but the buyer should beware that few web sites are static.

To further explore any of the Internet sites included in this list of references, copy the URL address and paste it into your browser.

Ref #	Title	URL
1	New to Type 1 Diabetes?	http://www.joslin.org/new_to_type_1_diabetes_information_for_parents.html
2	A Child You Care About Has Type 1 Diabetes	http://web.diabetes.org/wizdom/download/parents.asp
3	Coming to terms with your child's diabetes diagnosis	http://www.diabetes.co.uk/diabetes-and-parenting.html
4	Anne and John	http://www.childrenwithdiabetes.com/parents/d_03_1di.htm
5	Blue Christmas	http://www.childrenwithdiabetes.com/parents/d_03_1cy.htm
6	Parents of Children Newly Diagnosed with Type 1 Diabetes May Feel Lost, Alone...	http://diabetesadvocates.org/parents-of-children-newly-diagnosed-with-type-1-diabetes-may-feel/
7	Type 1 diabetes	http://www.diabetes.org/diabetes-basics/type-1/
8	What is type 1 diabetes?	http://www.diabetesresearch.org/what-is-type-one-diabetes
9	Type 1 diabetes facts	http://jdrf.org/about-jdrf/fact-sheets/type-1-diabetes-facts/
10	Type 1 diabetes: How is it treated?	http://kidshealth.org/teen/diseases_conditions/growth/treating_type1.html#
11	Type 1 Diabetes: Children Living With the Disease - Treatment Overview	http://www.webmd.com/diabetes/tc/type-1-diabetes-children-living-with-the-disease-treatment-overview
12	Type 1 diabetes	http://health.usnews.com/health-conditions/diabetes/type-1-diabetes/treatment
13	Type 1 Diabetes: Children Living With the Disease - Treatment Overview	http://www.webmd.com/diabetes/tc/type-1-diabetes-children-living-with-the-disease-treatment-overview
14	Islet cells and other strange things:	http://isletcellsandotherstrangethings.blogspot.com/search?updated-max=2012-07-09T00:29:00-07:00&max-results=7
15	We're asking the wrong question	http://liliesandlions.blogspot.com/search?updated-max=2012-04-28T19:06:00-07:00&max-results=7
16	My Child Has Diabetes	http://www.healthcentral.com/diabetes/just-diagnosed-411-143.html
17	When your child is diagnoses with a	https://www.apa.org/helpcenter/chronic-illness-child.aspx

	chronic illness: How to cope	
18	When a Child is Diagnosed with Type 1 Diabetes	http://www.aboutkidshealth.ca/en/resourcecentres/diabetes/understandingthediagnosisofdiabetes/pages/when-a-child-is-diagnosed-with-type-1-diabetes.aspx
19	Parents. Type 1 diabetes	https://www.bd.com/resource.aspx?IDX=22109
20	Care of Children and Adolescents With Type 1 Diabetes.	http://care.diabetesjournals.org/content/28/1/186.full.pdf
21	Overview of Diabetes in Children and Adolescents	http://ndep.nih.gov/media/youth_factsheet.pdf
22	Care of Children and Adolescents With Type 1 Diabetes. A statement of the American Diabetes Association.	http://care.diabetesjournals.org/content/28/1/186.full#sec-3
23	The Care Team	http://www.lvhn.org/conditions_treatments/diabetes/type_1_diabetes_overview/the_care_team
24	Care suggestions	http://www.childrenwithdiabetes.com/clinic/care.htm
25	Helping Your Child or Teen Live with Type 1 Diabetes	http://jdrf.org/life-with-t1d/type-1-diabetes-information/control-and-management/helping-your-child-or-teen-live-with-type-1-diabetes/
26	Psychological issues in the care of children and adolescents with type 1 diabetes	http://www.ncbi.nlm.nih.gov/pmc/articles/PMC2720894/
27	Psychological issues in the care of children and adolescents with type 1 diabetes	http://www.ncbi.nlm.nih.gov/pmc/articles/PMC2720894/
28	The 600-Step Program for Type 1 Diabetes Self-Management In Youth: The Magnitude of the Self-Management	http://www.andrews.edu/sed/gpc/faculty-research/coffen-research/coffen_2009_600.pdf

29	The 600-Step Program for Type 1 Diabetes Self-Management In Youth: The Magnitude of the Self-Management Task	http://www.andrews.edu/sed/gpc/faculty-research/coffen-research/coffen_2009_600.pdf
30	Helping Your Child Manage Type 1 Diabetes	http://health.cvs.com/GetContent.aspx?token=f75979d3-9c7c-4b16-af56-3e122a3f19e3&chunkiid=41883
31	Changing Patterns of Self-Management in Youth with Type I Diabetes.	http://www.sciencedirect.com/science/article/pii/S0882596306000741 (Abstract only)
32	Helping Your Child or Teen Live with Type 1 Diabetes	http://jdrf.org/life-with-t1d/type-1-diabetes-information/control-and-management/helping-your-child-or-teen-live-with-type-1-diabetes/
33	How to Deal With the 'Diabetes Police'	http://diabeteshealth.com/read/2005/10/01/4367/how-to-deal-with-the-diabetes-police/
34	How Friends, Coworkers Can Turn Into the Diabetes Police	http://www.health.com/health/condition-article/0,,20189188,00.html
35	Diabetes etiquette for parents. What your teen would like you to know	Card available at: www.behviioraldiabetes.org.
39	How Your Family and Friends Can Help You Manage Your Diabetes	http://www.onetouch.com/articles/relationshipstwo
37	Diabetes myths	http://www.diabetes.co.uk/diabetes-myths.html
38	Diabetes Myths	http://www.diabetes.org/diabetes-basics/myths/
39	Myths and Facts About Type 1 Diabetes	http://jdrf.org/life-with-t1d/type-1-diabetes-information/myths-and-facts/
40	Caregiver Stress Syndrome	https://www.vmvhypoallergenics.com/skintelligencenter/lifestyle/416-caregiver-stress-syndrome-living-with-children-with-allergic-conditions
41	Exhaustion, anger of caregiving get a name	http://comfortdoc.squidoo.com/caregiver-syndrome

42	Managing Caregiver Burnout When a Child has Diabetes. Taking care of your child while you take care of yourself.	http://type1diabetes.about.com/od/childrenwithtype /a/Managing-Caregiver-Burnout-When-A-Child-Has-Diabetes.htm
43	Managing Caregiver Burnout When a Child has Diabetes. Taking care of your child while you take care of yourself	http://type1diabetes.about.com/od/childrenwithtype /a/Managing-Caregiver-Burnout-When-A-Child-Has-Diabetes.htm
44	Tips for Coping With Caregiver Stress	http://www.webmd.com/balance/stress-management/caregiver-advice-cope
45	Caregiver Tip Sheet	: http://www.strokecamp.org/content/resourcesCAR/C aregiverTipSheet.pdf
46	Parents and Chronic Illness	http://www.parents.com/parenting/better-parenting/advice/parents-and-chronic-illness/?page=1
47	Adjusting Expectations to Meet the Reality of Diabetes. Be Kind to Yourself: Don't Expect Perfection	http://www.diabeticconnect.com/diabetes-information-articles/general/286-adjusting-expectations-to-meet-the-reality-of-diabetes
48	Extinguishing Burnout	http://www.diabetesselfmanagement.com/articles/ki ds-and-diabetes/extinguishing-burnout/print/
49	Perfection, Diabetes Don't Mix	http://www.diabetesselfmanagement.com/Blog/Davi d-Spero/perfection-diabetes-dont-mix/
50	Diabetes Challenges: Pursuing Perfection	http://www.healthadvisor.com/post/diabetes/diabet es-challenges-pursuing-perfection
51	Life expectancy improves for type 1 diabetics	http://usatoday30.usatoday.com/news/health/medic al/health/medical/diabetes/story/2011/06/Life-expectancy-improves-for-type-1-diabetics/48851072/1
52	Life Expectancy Increasing for Type 1 Diabetics, According to Latest Pitt Research	http://www.upmc.com/media/newsreleases/2012/pa ges/life-expectancy-increasing-type-1-diabetics.aspx
53	Life Expectancy Greatly Improved in Type 1 Diabetes.	http://www.medscape.com/viewarticle/811610#1